The Kids Are Grown, Now What?

Before you know it :)

A Guide for Couples to Touch & Reconnect

Angela Dunston Thomas

*Travis + Jessica
Be Blessed!*

*Enjoy
Angela Thomas*

ISBN-13:978-1984096265
ISBN-10:1984096265

Dedication

I dedicate this book first and foremost to God, my Light and my Salvation. To my husband, Alan, for his love, patience and friendship, as we learn to live in our empty nest and enjoy being connected to each other. To my mother, Rev. McBride, I love you mama! My girls, Toni, Teena and Jae, I love you to the moon and back! Thank you to my sisters and brothers, for always supporting me with your love and encouragement. To all my single and married friends, who shared their stories, fears and victories with me. To my cheering squad who stood firm with me from the beginning; a big THANK YOU to Anthony & Tonglia Davis, Tammy Griffin-Davis, Jennifer Stoner, Barbara Gary, Cynthia Reese, LaVon & Michelle Thomas, E. Renee Davis, Rosalind Pressley, and Sherry Burke. Last but certainly not least, my prayer partners, Pastors' Michael & Ayakao Watkins, Tiffany Purifoy, Iris Williams, Ray & Dorothy Raver and Doretha Jackson. This has been a journey, and I could not have done this without you Tina!

Contents

Foreword

To my sister and dear friend Angela, the definition of "Pride" is "A feeling or deep pleasure or satisfaction derived from one's own achievements or the achievements of those with whom one is closely associated." This word is so appropriate, because I'm filled with overwhelming "Pride" to be able to say this amazing woman is my sister and my best friend! I am also extremely "Proud" to see the amazing work that God has done in and through her! Angela has the biggest heart of anyone I know and she is always willing to open her heart and give love to those around. God has given her the gift of massage and through that gift He has allowed her to have and share her wisdom and insight on having a strong Godly marriage. Angela, I love you and Al with all my heart and I'm so grateful to be a part of this amazing journey! May God keep you and bless you more than you can ask or think!

With Love and Admiration, Your Sister, Tonglia Davis

Introduction

We began to ask God "now what?" The kids are grown, how do we reconnect as a couple? We really like each other and want to spend quality time together, not just live in the same house, where do we begin? We discovered, when couples try something new, they feel more attracted to each other. We started volunteering, sharing our hobbies, and traveling to places we had only dreamed of. Now we can spend more time with our family and friends. We enrolled in enrichment classes and re-enrolled in college to finally complete that degree. The best part was going on regular dates with each another.

This book is designed to support couples through the *empty nest* season where you can be refilled with expectations of excitement. You will become intentional through touch and continue to share meaningful love with your spouse. The goal is to reap the pleasure and desire God has promised in your marriage covenant. Many empty nests today are refilled with adult children and extended visits from grandkids and kinfolks. However, it is important to remember you are team one.

Chapter One

My Story, My Journey

The Will of God will never take you where the
Grace of God will not protect you.

~Billy Graham

As a young mom, fresh out of high school, I had the tremendous responsibility of raising a daughter. I soon found out it took a lot to provide a stable home and a peaceful environment. Me and her daddy were high school sweethearts. We met when we were 13 years old. We reconnected years later when we both reached dating age. Who would have thought that his life would be cut short? We had our whole lives to discover life and watch our daughter become a woman.... but unfortunately, after a brief illness, he died when he was only 35. He never got to see our daughter attend her prom, she was 16.

I grew up in a home with my mom, three brothers, two older, one younger. I also had a step-dad; until alcoholism consumed his life. Dad never had the chance to attend our younger brother's high school graduation. When our oldest brother joined the military, my 16-year-old God-sister moved in with us. Her mom died after a battle with cancer at the age of 35.

Growing up together as teenage girls, we were like two peas in a pod. The two of us were closer than most sisters for as long as I can remember. We spent a lot of time together since our parents were lifelong friends. She was only a few months older than me; she thought she was the boss. Our daughters were born only six months apart. We loved and cared like sisters; we even fought like sisters. We were not afraid to be honest with each other; we knew our sisterly love was genuine. My sister joined her mother in heaven when she was only 35, because of a tragic car accident.

The unhappiness I felt... it still rips my heart into pieces, even to think about it.

These were times of darkness where I felt absolutely lost, alone and sad. I felt like death had stolen too many people from my life, so quick, so fast. I was left numb, and nearly lifeless. I could hardly breathe. I felt like my life was operating on auto-pilot. I did the same things over and over, day after day, without any thought, went to work, came home, went to sleep, did it all over again. I was depressed but managing my day-to-day routine, going through the motions. I now realize God was carrying me through that darkness. I am forever grateful He brought me back into His marvelous sunshine to fully live again.

As a young mom, I grew, matured and practiced what I learned from my parents, grandparents, siblings, cousins, aunts and uncles; people I fondly refer to as "the Village." My village was the ladies in the neighborhood, teachers, church folks, corner store ladies, my friends' parents and any other adults my family was familiar with and respected. If "the village" saw me doing something out of line or me out of place, somehow without the use of cell phones, the word got back to my mother before I did. I learned the importance of love and respect from "the village." Lessons, both good and bad, were encountered while growing up in the Cove, where everybody knows everybody. When I heard, "is that little Angie, or does your mama know where you are?" I did not dare respond because my answer would be, she knows now! You know I said this in my head; out of respect, and honestly, out of fear of what would happen to me if I appeared to be disrespectable to adults.

In the South, we had several different names of affection for our mothers, such as Madea, Mom, Our Mama, and Mommy, just to name a few. We called our mother, Mama; she is a fantastic woman, and I would not trade her for any other, EVER. My mama is smart, caring, forgiving, and hard-working with strong faith in the Lord. Mama modeled and taught me countless skills and valuable lessons, which includes my unwavering trust in God. None of these lessons came easy for mama; she struggled and suffered through numerous trials and tribulations for what is now her greatest testimony. When she is teaching and preaching she knows God to be her Healer, Deliverer, Provider, Savior, Father, Mother, Sister, Brother, and Friend. I know her list does not stop there for who God is in her life. Rev. Mama is never ashamed to share the Good News of the Lord.

As I began to heal from the sadness, hurt, loss and loneliness, the Lord sent me an angel. I received a friend to walk by my side, to hold my hand, to hear my heart and respect my silence. His patience was like no other I had experienced in any relationship. I now have a friend that makes me laugh till I cry, let's me talk, be goofy, and just be me. I feel alive and restored with him by my side, giving me support and strength.

After a "long, long, long, time," as he puts it, he brought up the idea of us getting married, "since we have so much fun together" was his rationale. I thought, "oh no, there goes the fun!" I cannot take any more heartache, was shouting inside my head. I remembered trying that relationship path, and it did not turn out well for me. I said out loud in a sarcastic tone, "I'm good!" I thought, Lord, I do not want to mess up a perfectly good friendship! He kept being awesome and a great friend, the best in the world! He brought up the marriage idea again, later, much later. This time with major re-enforcement from my pastor, okay, yes! It took me a minute to really get it; my friends said, thank God, he was patient and persistent; hey, don't judge me! It took me a while to trust relationships and stop letting fear destroy my happiness. Yes, we finally got married, this was one of the best decisions I have ever made. My husband thought I had changed my mind when I was an hour late for the ceremony. He told me later my pastor calmed his fears by saying, "you know how she is, oh, she will be here." I'm still not clear on "how I am," but I love them both, and they love me.

Through the years I have had many experiences that have shaped me into who and what I am today. These decisions have taken me on many interesting and exciting journeys. I have been employed with the school system for nearly 30 years and worked in several districts. The importance of education was demonstrated throughout my family since most of my relatives work in the education field or has since retired from that arena.

The school system has been one adventure after another. Just in the first fifteen years, I have:

- been held hostage (by a chemically imbalanced co-worker);
- coached a talented cheerleading squad;
- dressed as a witch for Halloween;
- danced and chaperoned at prom and;
- helped deliver a baby.

Again, I will say this was just the first 15 years! I am thankful for all the lessons, the friends I have met, the places I have been, and the trials and blessings I have encountered throughout each chapter.

Chapter Two

Massage is My Therapy

"I've learned that every day you should reach out and touch someone. People love a warm hug, or just a friendly pat on the back."

~ Maya Angelou

The pain of sudden loss and the dreadful grip of grief pushed me into a place of sadness where I had to step back and exhale. There was never a good time to not work and concentrate on me, but now I needed a break. I was an emotional wreck. I had no choice; I had to get healthy and whole again. Only then would I be able to help anyone.

The Bondage Breaker author, Neil T. Anderson, stated that "we should treat emotional problems both physically and spiritually. There is no inner conflict which is not psychological because there is never a time when your mind, emotions and will are not involved. Similarly, there is no problem which is not spiritual. There is no time when God is not present or when it is safe for you to take off the armor of God."

During this break, I decided to become a full-time student, while our youngest daughter was a senior in high school. I had the love of family and friends for support and guidance. Our oldest daughter had married and started a family, and our middle daughter was enlisted in the United States Air Force. Many changes had taken place in our family.

The massage therapy course seemed interesting, and the class would take less than a year to complete, therefore, I registered. The date came for my orientation and testing. Everything went great, I passed the fundamentals. On the first day of class, the room was full of 20 something-year-old students. I thought to myself; this is going to be interesting. The teacher looked like he was around my age, and he immediately confirmed my thoughts by announcing his age to the class. Okay, now I am older than the teacher, great! I made it through the first day without having a panic attack. The students were very friendly and respectable. They referred to me as Miss Angie.

That evening while sharing my first day of school experience, I asked my husband, "What in the world did I get myself into?" Here I was 50 years old; I have been out of school for many years. I'm not sure I want to be with these young... okay, "young adults," I have a few "young adults" at home, and a break from them is paradise. Do they want me in their class; will they think I am like their mother? I started questioning myself, am I smart enough, will I pass this course, am I too old to do this? I was making a mountain out of a molehill. It was not that serious! They didn't care one way or the other; it was me who was tripping! Relax, Breathe, and Live in the moment! I had to do something to get me out of the sadness that was taking over my life.

Nevertheless, I made the commitment, and I had to be willing to put everything into the class to be successful. I must study, take great notes and practice. There was no way I would let these kids see me fail! Ha! The decision to take this course was a great decision even with all my unnecessary drama. I excelled in all my classes which included:

- Human Science;
- Anatomy & Physiology;
- Ethics & Business Law;
- Alignment & Movement;
- CPR & First Aid;
- Nutrition, Medication & Research; and
- Massage and Bodywork Techniques.

I was in class every day, received perfect attendance and served as the Class Ambassador. I took the examination to get licensed, and received my certification through National

Certification Board for Therapeutic Massage & Bodywork (NCBTMB). I have been performing therapeutic bodywork in the Atlanta Metro area for the last decade.

During the massage therapy course, I discovered several meanings of life's purpose and position. When you are facing unsettled times, God has a way of redirecting your heart to a path of healing for someone else that is going in that same direction. The decision to take the class and become a massage therapist was not just for my healing. It was for *His Glory* to help heal and reconnect couples who will find themselves in a nest that is empty and silent. I became a therapist to guide couples through massage touch as they reconnect with each other.

Now years later, and with three grown daughters, we get to enjoy dating each other again as empty nesters. We are beginning our second *Spring of Love* and we're determined to enjoy this new chapter in our relationship, and our lives. Our oldest granddaughter is in college, and with five other grandchildren growing fast, we pray they will follow her educational path.

We are willing as a couple to put in the effort as we grow and discover how to stay connected. We will continue to share our love and our time with family and friends. The couples who honor their spouse and learn to touch and communicate as they reconnect are discovering how to be satisfied in their empty nest.

Mike and Marilyn Phillipps, Founding Directors of Married for Life; the *Life-giving principles that make a marriage last;* stated, *"Marriage was intended by God to be a vibrant, dynamic state of ever-deepening love and growth. With God's direction, we can truly go from 'glory to glory' in our life together as husband and wife."*

Chapter Three

What's an Empty-Nest anyway?

"Just when I think I have learned the way to live, life changes."

~Hugh Prather

Being busy with life, the everyday hustle and bustle, the schedules of your jobs, your faith, family, friends, hobbies, marriages, deaths, and births, it may take a few years to realize your nest is empty. You may say, "we really are empty-nesters now! It happened so fast; they were just teenagers learning to drive, going to prom, graduation, wow, where did the time go?" You know that feeling I'm talking about, or you will soon find out, if you are heading in this direction.

Do not wait until your last child is on the way out of the house to begin preparing for your empty nest. Your goal is to raise healthy adults that will someday leave your home and live successful lives on their own. Get emotionally ready, when they are young; you will be better prepared for this season when the time comes, for you and for them.

Welcome to this new chapter of marriage. The Empty Nest! Having no children in the house can be a difficult transition for some parents. You probably thought you were prepared to be alone with each other before the kids left. This freedom from day to day parenting should be welcomed with great anticipation. After all, you can now go wherever you want, whenever you want and stay for as long as you like. The two of you probably started singing and dancing through the house in your underwear! It's now your time for romance and intimacy. Right!!??? It was more like "whatever!! We can now do nothing but rest and relax in our PJ's on the sofa, eating popcorn and M&M's, watching movies with the volume high.

It's our chance to leave the dishes in the sink, and sleep until noon."

As you started to look around it began to feel like the house was getting bigger, you barely saw each other or talked to each other. What was there to discuss, the kids are gone, and you can take care of yourself, you are adults. Your new freedom was beginning to feel like isolation! What was happening? You did not recognize the empty nest syndrome was moving into your space. You believed everything was going great, no one was complaining, at least not out loud. This was what you wished for when they were teenagers right? You always wanted peace and quiet, with a chance to do something for yourselves. After all, you are enjoying your own personal interests, hobbies, and TV shows. You have control of the remotes to your TVs, and the house is peaceful. What else is there, how can this be a problem?

Is this how it feels when it is just the two of you? Did the kids provide all your happiness? Did they keep you together as a family? Where are you headed? Are you getting old, too tired or just plain lazy? Maybe this is your time to exhale and rest from parenting all those years. After all, you need your space to unwind and rediscover the adults you are now.

You didn't know what was next. Something was not right, it was a disconnection. You shared fewer and fewer home-cooked meals together. No weekly trips to the grocery store. No real concern for health and wellness. You ate out at some nice restaurants, but still no real connection. Statistics show that couples age 50 and up are divorcing and experts say the trigger is often when their children leave home. But the reality is that years spent raising kids often turn parents into very different people from who you were when you got married. Now is the time to rediscover who you are as a couple.

Your kids are grown, how do you reconnect as a couple? You like each other and you want to spend more time together, not just live in the same house as roommates, how do you begin again? Where do you go from here, how do you start? When couples spend time, and do something new together, they feel more attracted to each other.

New statistics from the Office for National Statistics (ONS) states that couples could be waiting for their children to leave home before getting divorced. Lawyers also reported this after new figures showed the over-50 "silver separators" are the only age group in which divorce rates are rising.

This is your time to redefine yourselves as a married couple. Your empty nest involves challenges that can help you discover you are more than parents; you are a mighty team of one. Remember what it felt like to spend the nights on the lake fishing and skinny dipping? What about taking that salsa dance class, maybe now you have the patience to learn the steps! Now is your time to identify new roles and interests, while reviving existing activities you put on the back-burner while the kids were growing up. Make a list of who you are and what you do for yourself and others. Look at your roles; can you spend more time in these areas? Do you have new areas you are willing to discover? Mission trips are always great for couples who volunteer; maybe it is time you considered signing up, not only will you help others, you will also support yourself and your marriage.

Start serving outside the house by volunteering and sharing your hobbies with others, traveling to places you both planned to visit. Begin spending more time with others. Enroll in self-enrichment classes, or college to sharpen your skills. One of the best discoveries is going on regular dates. Dating is great, not to mention interesting during this chapter of your marriage.

Find out if your pilot light is still lit, but you must be intentional to turn up the heat. Marriage is like a fire; you must constantly rekindle it to keep it going. In her book; *Personality Plus for Couples: Understanding Yourself and the One You Love*; Florence Littauer writes, *"we fall in love with a person's strengths, but one day we wake up and realize we're married to their weaknesses!"* Healthy marriages are no accident.

Getting out of your comfort zone and doing something different may be uncomfortable as you begin the reconnection discovery. Be patient with each other, listen and hear suggestions with your heart as you step into this new world for you two. Mothers tend to have a harder time dealing with the children leaving than their husbands. With that in mind, stay in prayer and remember you are Team One!

You made a vow to work and pray at honoring the covenant you promised each other, God, and your families. It is heartbreaking when couples who have been married for decades, decide to separate after all they have invested in each other and their family. This dream killer must stop destroying families. Become aware why this is happening to marriages and pray you avoid these pitfalls.

Too many times we see couples outside, appearing so happy, smiling, wearing the happy masks for the world to see. But on the inside, it is a different story. You can be happy inside and out! It takes work; marriages do not run on auto-pilot. You said the kind words, did the nice things and put in the extra work at the beginning of your love story. It is time to rediscover that precious love! You know the importance of touching your spouse and the positive difference it makes in your relationship. Sometimes, you become slack in your efforts; now is your time to become more intentional with your loving embrace.

You have a responsibility to your spouse and to yourself to do the work it takes and show your children and grandchildren that marriage covenant and commitment is real, and it can work. Married life should be great inside together and outside with others. Marriages can last until death separates you. With God, **all** things are possible.

When you entered God's plan for marriage, you agreed that it became "we" and no longer just "me." Team One! As covenant partners, you also exchanged all that you both previously held separately. According to 1 Corinthians 7:4, even our bodies were given to each other. All our goods, our wealth, belong to each other jointly. God says that the two become one (Ephesians 5:3) and in covenant, everything belongs to the one.

Family life is a busy life and raising kids is a great responsibility for parents. However; it is not your entire life. There is life after the kids are grown. Take time and evaluate your lives as individuals and as a couple. Visualize the upgrades you now have around you.

Some of the upgrades of being empty nesters you didn't know existed until the kids were grown:

- **Your house is clean and everything in place**
  The kids' clothes, shoes, books, CDs, movies and other items are not scattered all over the house. The bathroom towels are clean and hanging neatly, the dishes are put away, beds are made, floors are clean, and clothes are out of sight. There are no mystery spills, and you never come home to a mess you did not create. You didn't know it could be this good!

- **It is quiet in the house**
  Shhhh.... did you hear that??? What??? Nothing, it's quiet. The sound level is peaceful in the house now that the television, radio and CD player are not all booming at the same time. You can actually hear yourself think.

- **You discover you still like each other**
  Remember why you fell in love in the first place. You are each other's company when you are home. Look at each other and say, "It is just us now, let's enjoy this time together and rediscover who we are.

- **You can sleep through the night**
  You are no longer waiting for the kids to come in the door, or turning off the porch light after they get home safe. You are not a part of their daily lives, no matter how many times they text and call you in a day. Their mental

and physical wellness is still important to you, but they are responsible now for themselves. You do not have to endure the worries of their daily lives like you did when they lived at home. You did a great job. Now it is time to let your young adults bloom.

- **Your food expenses are less**
Buy food and drinks you enjoy. Stock the pantry and refrigerator with items you like and that are good for your health. Preparing meals for two is less expensive and easier to plan.

- **Your cash on hand lasts longer**
You have extra cash in your wallet when you need it. You are not handing out money like it grows on trees. Your gas needle is where you left it.

- **You have free time to do more of what you enjoy**
You have discovered the pleasure of doing nothing; you are happy being in a quiet and clean home together. Enjoying one venture after another; attending concerts, movies, theater and traveling. Whatever it is, you have more time to do it.

- **You now spend time with people you enjoy being around**
You have great friends; now you have more time to spend with them. Schedule weekday and off-peak season trips with friends who are also empty nesters.

- **You spend time with your kids as young adults**
This is probably one of the most satisfying elements of being an empty nester. Your children leave home and, for better or worse, they grow up. It is a blessing seeing them as adults, taking charge of their lives and making decisions. You feel proud of your offspring, enjoy being with them as adults and allow them to enjoy their time with you.

- **Your kids come to visit**
  It is great seeing them after weeks or months away when you honestly miss them. Their faces are welcoming. Beautiful, warm, friendly smiles are all you need. It is such a thrill to have them home for holidays, summer, or just a weekend visit; and within minutes of their return, it is as if they never left. You love having them home for a while.

- **They return to their house**
  You love your empty nest.

- **Your future is yours**
  Remember when your world was extensive, and you had no idea what you were going to do next? Well, you can dream again, now that you are an empty nester. You have no worries about childcare, or kids missing school, or whether they will like the place you decide for vacation. It is your time, your future, and your life.

  You both have always wanted to travel around the world, now you can. Go back to school and expand your knowledge. Write that book; someone is waiting to read it, so get started. You have your lives to live, just as your kids have theirs. Start living the life you were created to live!

  "Your child's life will be filled with fresh experiences.
  It's good if yours is as well."
  ~Dr. Margaret Rutherford

Chapter Four

Maintain a Connection with the Kids

Live without pretending, love without depending,
listen without defending & speak without offending.
~Unknown

Being a parent to your adult children can be a challenge when you're trying to find the balance between being their friend, mentor and parent.

During this new season, you will explore the best options on how you communicate to keep a connection with them. Be the parents who talk *with* your children and not *at* them. You and your kids will learn how to stay in your own lane and mind your own business; simply respect one another.

The more you communicate with your kids about everyday situations, the easier it will be later, when more pressing issues come to the surface. Keep the lines of communication open for them to share with you just as they did when they were still at home. Talk with them often. Gentle guidance may help situations they may face as they grow and mature. Your kids always want to know you care, even when they don't show it.

I cannot stress this enough, keep the communication doors open between you and your children. Never leave them out, no matter how "grown" they are. Don't start giving them advice and suggestions when they are ready to leave the nest. It is an on-going process and your communication starts early in their lives.

It's difficult for them to accept your suggestions once they are out of the house if they struggled with this while living with you. Be gentle and honest; no one is perfect. Young adults do not always welcome and readily accept your advice, don't be offended. Wait for them to ask for your opinion before offering. Your children can make their own decisions, good or bad. Have faith; you did a great job parenting them. Relax; they are learning just as you did. Try not to be so quick to say, "I told you so, you should have listened to me." This will drive a wedge between you both, and it will be hard to remove and get them to listen again. When you communicate often, through email, text, phone calls, or in person, you will know something is wrong before they say it. That is being a parent.

When your children get into "a situation" and need help, whether you feel they made a right or wrong decision, be there for them. You are their safety net. There will be times they need you to simply listen. No matter how difficult things may appear, sometimes; let them work it out. Your kids will let you know when to step in and when to stay back. Allow them to learn and grow through their experiences.

James Dodson put it this way... "Children are not casual guests in our home. They have been loaned to us temporarily for loving them and instilling a foundation of values on which their lives will be built."

As parents of adult children, you can become anxious when it comes to your kids finding a soul mate. You may feel no one is good enough for your son or daughter. Well, parents beware, there are good men and women out there and your kids will find them. You may not see what they see, and it does not matter. It is their decision. Pray and trust your children. Trust they have the values and morals you instilled in them.

Be supportive of their decisions, do not always be critical. The world needs more love in families, especially when grandchildren come along. It is better to show love and live by example.

Showing your children love and respect throughout their growing years really pays off when they are grown. You begin to see the fruit of your labor, the morals you taught and modeled. Some kids need to discover who they are and the plan God has for their lives. What you see in them may not be the dream you saw for them. What you see is the test, to get them to their testimony. Trust God; He has the whole world in His hands. Stay connected to them in a positive way and continue to be their example.

"It is easier to build strong children than to repair broken men."
~Fredrick Douglass

Chapter Five

Dating with Flavor!

"Choose Life over the other stuff. Get out of your head. Live. Dress up. Eat. Touch people. Help out. Give up. Love people. Give your best away. There's more. What's the problem? Relax. You're going to die. Throw a party. Eat off my plate. Sing to me. Meet me in the bedroom. Get a massage. Give one. Let your amazement out into the room. Pry open the box you hide your joy in. Be a poem."
~John Patrick Shanley

Dating as a married couple gives you many opportunities to reconnect. You will share special times rekindling your flame at a much slower pace than what you had at your beginning.

Before you made the commitment to get married, you put on your best behavior. You impressed one another with gifts, compliments, talents and listened to each other. You took extra time preparing for your date, making sure everything was perfect. You made reservations to special places and you were on time. You impressed your friends and family with your new "boo" and boasted about how happy you were to have them in your life. The two of you talked and talked for hours, sharing hopes and dreams of your future together. You created a bond of friendship as you shared your lives together.

This was the beginning of your romantic relationship, your friendship that began with a promise. Romance is friendship. In reading the Song of Solomon 5:16, Solomon praises his bride saying, *"This is my lover, this is my friend."* Now, at this stage in your relationship, you have discovered important details about each other and what *love language* your spouse speaks and needs. The book, *the 5 Love Languages* by Gary Chapman is a great book; if you don't know what *Love Language* your spouse speaks, this may be an excellent place to start. This tool can help you get on the same communication wave and effectively meet the needs of each other. Your *love language* can change over time, so it is best to re-evaluate how you're doing every now and then.

When couples in an empty nest begin to date again, it is rewarding to recognize you have been successful partners in nurturing your children into adulthood. You are at the sweet age; where you're still young enough to enjoy each other and old enough to have obtained a variety of experience in life lessons. Celebrate your marriage, and enjoy the best years with each other.

A date to the movies and sharing a meal is nice, if you haven't been on a date in a while, it's a start. Add some flavor to those dates, step it up, plan something unique and exciting that you both enjoy. Now if you're spending money to make yourself look good and checking off a box where you have met that obligation; please rethink your motives. Do not let your dates be another chore, live in the moment, be present. Give of yourself freely, and honestly. The commitment is powerful, it shows you care.

If you know he loves *Almond Joy* candy bars, you can send a movie date reminder with the candy bar or a picture of one! Put a card with movie tickets in the laptop bag with the candy bar. Send a rose with the movie tickets in a card. It's the little things that matter.

Surprising ways to say I love you are endless. Explore ventures you have talked about over the years. Be intentional. The key is to create memories you can share for years to come. Make your marriage a priority and learn to fall in love over and over and plan to be in love for life. Give your full attention to your lover by showing them you care and telling them they are important to you.

Make lists of places to visit, things to do and people to meet. Take turns selecting from the list, then let the exploration begin. Go back to some of the places and events you have already experienced; maybe it was with the kids, give it another visit, together. Take your time, smell the roses. Share your ideas with each other about planning time together. Developing a deep level of friendship through shared interests is one of the first ingredients in a romantic relationship.

Clear communication and shared details are important in planning dates. Attend the movies and bowling at midnight can be a fun night out. Or you can enjoy dinner at home; hire a chef to cook the meal. Order takeout and meet in the park for dinner after work. Go to an amusement park, visit the aquarium, become a tourist in your hometown. Get together and spend time getting to know who you are now in this stage of life and share your future together as an empty nest couple. Talk about how it feels to live in the house without the kids.

Relationships can get boring; things might become routine since we are creatures of habit, it is easy to do. So; spice it up, live and enjoy this life you have been given. Have fun scheduling the dates and spending time with each other. You will create memories and stories that will be exciting to share, even with your grandchildren. Celebrate birthdays, anniversaries and holidays in unique ways no one will ever forget. It feels good to be loved and know someone loves you back.

Balancing your time and sharing it with others can be both fun and challenging. Of course, your family wants you to be happy; your happiness and love will shine brightly for others to see. It is encouraging to observe older couples in love, holding hands and embracing in public and sharing loving kisses and hugs. Long-time married couples are often asked how their marriages survived after their children grew up. Most couples said they continued to spend quality time together. Honor and respect were also mentioned as assets for their happy homes.

After listening to these couples about what worked to keep them connected. One husband said his wife is, "the best cook in the world, and as sure as cornbread goes with greens, she is the answer to his dreams!" Now from this southern girl's point of view;

he promises to be with her forever! Another couple mentioned they always keep the lines of communication open between them. They said, simply, "we honor and respect each other." When the couples talked about their empty nest experiences; they put each other first, before their children, so when their kids left they still had that bond with one another.

It was clear; the simple things in life are the most important. Schedule regular dates. There will be times when plans don't go as scheduled. *Try* and keep on *trying*. If you're the one who has always made the arrangements, maybe now is the time to let it go. Learn to be open-minded, let your hair down, try something different. Listen and be willing to get out of the box and trust your date. You may be pleasantly surprised. This could be the spark you need to restart the flame.

- Communicate with each other when planning a date to avoid conflicts.

- Be aware of pitfalls when scheduling your time together.

- Watch for hidden interruptions.

- Make your date a priority. You are worth it.

- If you cancel, reschedule your date immediately.

- Do not allow other people's poor planning to interfere with your schedule.

Be spontaneous every now and then, remember the kids are grown! Do not get stuck doing the same old thing over and over! Routines take out the sparkle; then the date becomes a duty. The goal is to enjoy each other, have fun, and be intentional. Marriage takes prayer and faith in action. Do your part, make it last!

Dating ideas used when planning your time together. Do not limit yourself or your imagination. The sky is the limit, go for it!

Go dancing	Take a hot air balloon ride
Go hiking	Take a class
Drive a race car	Go to the aquarium
Pose for pics in a photo booth	Attend a concert
Attend Bible Study	Volunteer at a shelter
Work at the food bank	Cook with friends
Schedule a couple's photo shoot	Get *Massages*
Watch the sunrise	Watch the sunset
Go for a walk	Go to a bookstore
Enjoy a candlelight dinner	Babysit

"Do what makes you happy
Be with who makes you smile
Laugh as much as you breathe
And love as long as you live."
~Earl Dibbles Jr.

To bring passion back into your marriage, take this *kissing challenge*. Kiss each other for about 15 seconds each day. Do not start counting the seconds; just be in the moment long enough for a lingering passionate kiss that says I will marry you all over again.

Well, until we took this challenge, our kissing became routine like so many other things in our life. This kissing challenge has been around for years. There are books written on it, and people talking about it.

In this challenge, it tells *a story about a young man who had been married for several years. His wife was incredible, his kids were awesome, and things were going well for them. For the most part, his marriage was good, but there was a disconnection. The passion was gone, and he didn't know why. One day he decided to bring up the topic of marriage to his dad. If anyone had a great marriage, it was his parents. Married for over 30 years, they still held hands and always smiled at each other like teenagers in love.*

"Dad, what is your secret?" he asked, "Why is your marriage so strong, when so many others are failing?" Taking off his watch, he passed it to his son, who turned it around to read the inscription. "15 seconds every day ~ no less." "I got this watch from my father," he said, "and now I am giving it to you. Kiss her 15 seconds every day. No less. Come back to me in a month and tell me if it does not make a difference."

Let me tell you, after I heard this *story*, I wondered; could 15 seconds *really* make a difference? I had to try it out in my laboratory (the kitchen), and my handsome "boo" just happened to be near. Approaching him for a kiss, I leaned in. He responded with the usual quick peck on the lips, but just as he started to slip away, I grabbed his waist, pulled him in close and whispered, "Let's try that again, but longer." 15 seconds was all it took for the passion to wash over me, reminding me of how I fell deeply and passionately in love with him.

Who knew that one little kiss could make such a big difference? Apparently, King Solomon did when he wrote these beautiful words in Song of Solomon 1:2, *"Let him kiss me with the kisses of his mouth: for your love is better than wine."*

Chapter Six

Words are Powerful

"Use what talents you possess; the woods would be very silent if no birds sang there except those that sang best." ~Henry Van Dyke

Words are powerful. We are not going down the path where we speak negative, hurtful and insensitive words. We will take the high road where we build each other up with encouraging words. Meaningful communication makes your heart smile. It is comforting to be in the presence of someone who says kind and encouraging words that give you honor and respect. We all know how good encouragement feels. Without added kindness, a marriage will suffer.

Do you remember when you first met? You talked and talked for hours at a time. You talked about everything and then about nothing, and somehow, you loved every minute of it. As the years went by, the kids did all the talking. Now it's you again. Wow, it's strange you don't have much to say! What in the world happened? Now is the time to get the fuel and restart the flame of communication. Be intentional in having regular conversations with your spouse. Conversations can begin in the morning while getting dressed, during the day while at work, at lunchtime, after work, during dinner, before bed and during your prayer time together.

Began saying nice and encouraging words to your spouse every day. A great start is to begin with a few simple words such as "good morning honey, have a great day, and see you later." Always speak in a cheerful and pleasant tone. Don't take each other so seriously, it is a necessity to laugh and be playful with one another; this is a great way to communicate. When you experience a rough patch, or feel stressed; do not destroy your mate with your tone of voice, silence or with no expression of interest. Choose your words wisely. If you have verbalized something you wished you could take back, apologize, ask God and your partner to forgive you, then both of you move forward.

Praying together is another way to build firm blocks of communication. Share your fears and victories with each other. Remember you are a team. Listening with understanding is powerful and this alone can save you from being misunderstood. If you feel your message wasn't received in the spirit you said it and your partner took offense to your words, take a moment to clarify what you meant, explain it until you both comprehend. This does not say you will always agree. It means you understand each other. Clear it up when things are foggy between you; do not let it gnaw at your bond.

Communication is important in every relationship. It is the cement that holds it together or the sand that grinds it apart. We must be reminded not to talk all the time. Watch what you say, and practice being a good listener. Do not be afraid of the silence; this can be refreshing. It has been said that, silence is golden. Sometimes it's best to be silent and think before you say something you cannot take back. However, silence is not the way to solve problems; you must work through them with effective communication skills. Sharing your day and life with each other will certainly help you stay linked.

Practice being intentional as you communicate and getting to know each other again.

- Your eyes express love and approval. Be sure your heart is also showing your passion and not just your words alone.

- Give your loving smile to your spouse every day. Speak encouraging words with praise and acceptance.

- Be kind and thankful. Good manners and being courteous goes a long way.

- Always kiss hello and goodbye to release the love hormone, Oxytocin; this creates an environment for trust, respect, safety, and love.

- Thirty-second hugs are simple and powerful; they can bring you closer to each other. These small embraces can translate into a deeper emotional connection.

These actions speak volumes. They will come naturally as you reveal them every day with your lover. You will remember how good it felt when your love was young and fresh. The vows you made to each other, to love, honor and cherish; has ushered you into this precious moment in your marriage, enjoy this gift.

Chapter Seven

Your Mind Right & Your Body Tight

"He who has health, has hope; and he who has hope, has everything."   ~Thomas Carlyle

During the empty nest years, many changes can take place in your body and your mind. These changes can be challenging. While trying to keep pace with your job, parents, children, hobbies, and spouse; exercise is a must. Your health can be attacked physically by illnesses or accidents. We do not plan for these unforeseen circumstances, they just show up. Regular fitness routines can help you recover better, faster.

Good physical health is a significant component to living an active lifestyle, along with mental clarity to help guide your decisions. Do not ignore the care you give yourself. Let your loved ones see you taking good care of yourself. Eat healthier meals, get proper sleep and regular health checkups. Remember if you ignore your health it will go away!

God designed us with a Central Nervous System (CNS) which consists of three parts, motor nerves, autonomic nerves and sensory nerves. The Sensory nerves; which transmit pain to your body; is a small part compared to the other section of the CNS. You could feel healthy and something could be wrong. Even though you are feeling good and functioning day-to-day, something inside of your body could be suffering. Waiting for pain to signal you to visit your doctor can be harmful to your health. It is essential to get regular checkups to help avoid major problems later. Do not wait for the pain.

Learn to relax and minimize the stress in your life. Be careful of those who rob you of your happiness. As you already know and have experienced by now, people, even those who love us, can steal our joy. Their problems can become our problems if we're not careful. Remember you are a couple and the two of you can handle situations more skillfully. Your load is much lighter when it is divided. Trust in your faith and always know help is only a prayer away. You are never alone. None of us can live this life without our creator guiding us and supporting us when we need help.

Keep in mind, this is a new road for the two of you. Walk it together, talk about the changes and share your thoughts with the one you are connected to for life. Be attentive to your partner and provide support that shouts, I LOVE, HONOR AND RESPECT YOU!

Living at home without kids really changes the dynamics of your life. It is a good thing. Preparing meals is new for both of you as empty nesters. Food preparation is an excellent aphrodisiac. Be adventurous with meals and meal planning; try foods you have never tasted. Switch things around. Enjoy having your breakfast meal for dinner. Experiment with different foods to heighten your sense of taste and smell. Join a cooking class and learn new techniques and skills. Host a class with your family and friends; practice your new cooking skills. Experiment with old and new recipes and include ingredients that are new to you.

Fellowship with friends, family or your neighbors for a seven-course meal. Enjoy each course at a different house. Until you get to the dessert, have that course at home! It can be stimulating to change your dining scene every now and then. Eat outside on the patio, pack a dinner basket and eat in the park. Get your gear and go fishing and cook your catch on the lake. Enjoy a seafood feast on the beach. Remember you have the freedom to cook what and how you want, live it up!

This is your time to pamper yourselves with manicures, pedicures, facials, and massages. This helps you reconnect by experiencing these relaxing sessions together. Enroll in classes such as dancing, swimming, belly-dancing, golf, and tennis. Hang out and socialize with family and friends you have not seen in a while. Go on adventurous trips together to places you have only dreamed of visiting. Sign up and go on mission trips together.

Amusement parks are a blast when you revisit them as a couple. Go at your own pace; enjoy the attractions that interest you. Try different restaurants or prepare a picnic basket and enjoy it on the grounds. Take a break for a nap, or go window shopping. Have fun, laugh and play. Enjoy the journey.

Appreciating good food, and outside activities is necessary, but physical pleasure is a priority. A healthy sex life seems to contribute to a healthy immune system. Research suggests there is a positive link between sex and lower blood pressure. Now that's a great reason to stay active. Another reason why you should enjoy regular love making; its good exercise and you can burn 150 calories. You know exercise is good for your heart! Additional benefits of lovemaking; it improves your bladder control. Anatomy research has shown, for women, the Kegel pelvic floor muscles are being worked. This contributes to the tightening of your PC muscles as it relates to your bladder. The muscles are strengthened and provide support for the pelvic organs because of the physical motion and intensity. More and more reasons to stay connected; sex is healthy and relaxing, like a massage for the whole body. Intimate sexuality will deepen your spiritual bond with each other. Now, that is how God planned it!

Not only is spending time together valuable and important, to do that effectively, you must show up for yourself! You will gain mental clarity. Love on you! Do not fill all your time with others and forget about spending time with yourself, alone. Do whatever it is you care to do; major pampering, read a book, enjoy a movie, get a massage, visit friends, or work on your hobby. Balance is the key. You will be more loving and willing to share the best of you with those you love when you're able to spend time alone.

Remember the Great Commandment... Love God with all your heart, your soul, your mind, and all your strength. Here you see the four main areas that make us human, our *heart* (spiritual), *soul* (emotional), *mind* (intellectual) and *strength* (physical). Love yourself, take care of yourself and in your overflow, you can love and take care of others.

Chapter Eight

More Money Honey

Live a full life. The key to happiness is spending money on experiences instead of things.

~Unknown

Financial Planning is essential during this time of your marriage. Now is the time to re-focus on your goals and re-evaluate your financial muscle. Where are you headed from here? How do you plan to get there? Some things to consider are your spending habits, your retirement, long-term care options and maybe downsizing your current home.

No one wants to work until they die unless it is something you would do for free. The reality is that people have done just that. They have died on the job, never able to retire and enjoy life.

Your spending habits may change when it is just the two of you. Develop an Estate Plan to organize your financial records, assets, titles, and beneficiaries. Consider buying a vacation home, purchasing a new car or investing more into your retirement savings plan. This is a great time to explore your retirement options and plan an exit strategy from work.

Prepare a Will, and decide on a Power of Attorney for your assets. Draft a Health Directives Plan, which provides your instructions in case you are unable to speak for yourself. This is the time to have "the talk" and get your plans in black and white. It is great financial planning to have at least six months of income saved in case of an emergency.

During this season you may need to set financial boundaries with your children, extended family, and others. As a family you may decide to focus on your financial goals. It's a good plan if you need to save more money for retirement. Financial planning will certainly reduce stress and tension in your marriage through the golden years, resulting in more time to enjoy each other.

Ask yourself these questions. Now that the kids are grown, do you need that big house? Have you thought about getting a smaller place or relocating into an adult community? Make an appointment with your financial advisor and get a snapshot of your economic status. Now is the time to re-evaluate your savings and retirement plans to see if you are headed in the direction you planned many years ago when you began your careers. Did bad investments, illness, loss of job, debt or some other hardship cause a financial setback? How do you plan to bridge the financial gap? Do you need to work longer to maintain your current lifestyle? Will you retire and begin another career? These are some questions to consider when the two of you reach this season. Set new goals for your household. Strive for a credit-free life and a debt-free house.

Financial planning is making a sacrifice now to get greater gratification later. You will learn you don't need it all and you don't need it right now. *Dave Ramsey's, Financial Peace University Course*, provides detailed instructions on how to become debt free and avoid financial pitfalls. This is a great source for educating families on financial awareness. If you are in trouble, he has steps to help you get out and stay out. In his book, *Complete Guide to Money*, his motto is, *"If you live like no one else, later you can live like no one else."* He also stated, *"If you make some sacrifices, inject some discipline, and get intentional about winning with money, the future is wide open. You'll be blown away by the opportunities you'll have to serve and bless other people, and you'll be amazed at what life feels like without worrying about money all the time. It's a great place to be."*

There are several benefits when you start saving early and are intentional about your money, some examples are:
- The wedding expenses will not be shocking, and your kids can enjoy their big day.

- The opportunity for your child to study abroad is a reality.
- You can purchase a place on the beach.
- Retire and pursue your dreams.
- Sponsor missions and charities.
- Pay cash for your dream vehicle.
- Take the family on great vacations.
- Remodel your house, add that outdoor kitchen.
- Be debt free.
- Blessed to be a blessing.

- ✓ Remember to live within your means.
- ✓ Start saving early and invest wisely.

Unfortunate events that have caused families to lose everything and each other.
- He planned on retiring with 30 years of service, but got laid off with 27 years, with no pension, not even a watch. This is the reality many face in companies today.
- She had an accident at work and Workers Compensation only paid 60% of her salary. They have exhausted their savings account on living expenses.
- He was diagnosed with a disease; medical bills bankrupted the family.
- Their son needed a transplant; this depleted their entire retirement accounts.
- He has an addiction and rehabilitation hasn't helped.

- ✓ *You can recover when you are a team.*
- ✓ *But with God **all** things are possible.*

Chapter Nine

Just the Two of Us

"Shared joy is double joy; shared sorrow is half a sorrow."
                                                    ~Swedish Proverb

Now it's just the two of you. You have fewer interruptions and less stress in the home. Your schedules are carefully planned to add new experiences and your dates are anticipated with excitement. Protect your plans and make your dates a priority. Before you cancel or accept invitations or other projects, be sure it's in your best interest. It may seem easier to cancel your plans for someone or something else, but always ask each other these two questions:

1) Is this what's best for us?
2) Is it worth it to break our date?

Family members can pull you in different directions by planning events and extending invitations at the last minute. This can be unintentional on their part, but be aware. You may be able to avoid these emotionally draining situations from getting out of control by spending scheduled time with your kids, grandchildren, family, and friends.

Let those who love you, feel special too. Remember they are a big part of your life and they also help you survive. Enjoy the time you all share together. They miss their time with you as much as you miss them, so have fun when you're together. Your children will feel good by knowing their parents are doing well and getting along with each other. Seeing their parents happy makes them happy. You need each other, so pray daily for one another.

The responsibilities of the household chores are now shared between the two of you. This can be a fun adventure if you approach it with the right attitude, be creative. If the budget allows, hire someone to do this for you. It may be too much to handle, with all your planning and dating activities, who has time to clean?!

Today is the only gift of time you have been given. That's why it's called, the present. Use it wisely. Enjoy this new season to celebrate your love. Your empty nest will soon be your oasis when you put effort into making each other feel special, just as you did when you first met.

Share how you feel and remember to stick together as a team. Refocusing takes work, and marriage in an empty nest is a totally different and exciting chapter. The silence in the house can be awkward and feel strange in the beginning. Without the kids at home, you may see your spouse differently than you have in years. Reminisce the moments of your first dates together, when life was, *oh so simple*.

Being parents is an awesome responsibility. You are raising kids, giving directions, organizing everyone and everything, the list goes on and on. Mothers, sometimes have a harder time dealing with the transition to an empty nest than fathers, so it seems. Perhaps fathers do not readily admit they miss the kids as much as mom does, but they miss them too.

The mothers' role in the family is an important and busy one to say the least. She has been directing and correcting, while cooking and cleaning for the family. Now she finds herself alone in the house with her husband. Sometimes her words, actions and gestures, come across like a mom to her husband. She is giving orders, asking questions and providing the answers, all in the same breath. You have been mothering and nurturing children for so long it can be a difficult transition to change your mothers' voice and now just be a wife.

You may experience the loneliness of not having the children around, and feel your life is no longer needed as a mother. You may ask, now what? Be patient; meaningful conversation is still present in your marriage and you both will live, learn and adjust. Be patient as you rediscover the moments you decided to love each other for life. This is where the page turns, and your new chapter begins.

My lover and my friend. The most intimate time is when a couple is connected and they understand each other through gentle, vulnerable and non-sexual experiences. This happens when you enjoy spending time together. Here are some ways couples can enjoy the journey:

- Don't be so serious all the time. Be weird sometimes, laugh a lot, have fun!

- Marriage is a journey, not a destination. You are never going to get there, so enjoy the journey.

- Don't take things personally when one of you laughs. Nothing is wrong. Be open to give and take a joke. Tease and poke fun, all in the name of love. You would never intentionally hurt, harm or cause pain to someone you love and care about.

- Playfulness and laughing is a huge role in how you and your partner interact with each other.

- Light-heartedness releases chemicals in the brain that naturally put you in a better mood to give and receive love.

- Living in a house together and not effectively communicating with each other can make the house one of the loneliest places to be in.

- Create routines you look forward to doing together. Enjoy and experience life while making memories and adding new stories to share.

- Be comfortable around each other, naked. Do not be shy about your body. Be secure and confident.

- Everyone must change; no one stays the same! Yes, this also refers to your physical bodies, we all change. You may wake up and not recognize your own legs, arms or face, and maybe other body parts. It's like the invasion of the body snatchers!

- This is your lifelong partner that promised to be with you until the end. Hold them to it!

- Sharing time doing literally nothing can be comfortable and satisfying. Embrace the space.

- Laugh at your quirky inside jokes.

- There is no pretense in your interactions, you don't have to try hard with each other, your fun comes naturally.

- You are comfortable expressing bodily functions around each other; excuse me; yes, like belching and passing gas. You survived childbirth it's better out than in.

- Sometimes in life, the most basic human things can be the funniest.

- The couples that laugh together realize they don't mind being basic, hilarious and human.

These are the couples that have found the key to real happiness. It is simple, be yourself, love yourself, love God and then you can freely love your spouse.

Giving and serving others often promotes spiritual closeness in a marriage relationship. Use your time, talent and treasure to enrich the lives of others. You will experience joy and satisfaction in return. By mentoring young couples, both of you will learn something. Spend time with them and share your experiences, and wisdom by giving them encouragement and support in their relationships.

Fellowship and worshipping with others who share your beliefs will refill your nest with opportunities to serve and offer your wisdom. Focus on others; ask yourselves, what is God calling us to do together? How can our lives make a positive difference in others?

Explore your dreams and passions. Write them down; put your purpose in motion. Now is the time for your hopes and expectations to take flight, make it a mission you can pursue together. Studies by *Fincham & Beach* published in the *Journal of Family of Psychology, 2014*, suggested that couples who pray together describe their marriage as being *highly romantic*. The Journal also stated that *"couples who pray together regularly enjoy lovemaking more."* Studies show that couples who worship together have high levels of marital satisfaction and even higher levels of commitment to each other and their marriage covenant.

Instead of creating separate dreams, be a team. Find out what is unique about you. What are your values? What are you passionate about? Always ask God for wisdom and allow Him to guide you in ways that go beyond your plans and dreams. You will never be without a plan and a promise. Be patient; there is no time limit, no deadlines, enjoy each moment.

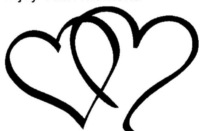

Chapter Ten

Intentional Touching

*"Love is patient, love is kind, and is not jealous;
love does not brag and is not arrogant, does not
act unbecomingly; it does not seek its own [will], is
not provoked, does not take into account a wrong
suffered, does not rejoice in unrighteousness, but
rejoices with the truth; bears all things, believes all
things, hopes all things, endures all things."*

~Paul the Apostle

Do you know how to touch effectively? Learning how to touch is essential. Touching is a skill for the most part; it has been forgotten and replaced with other activities. Do not assume because you're beautiful, handsome, smart, employed and have a great body you are the complete *package*. To compliment your *package*, learn the art of touch. It's a desired asset. Unfortunately, failure to understand this can open the door for you or your partner to seek the attention of others who have mastered this skill. This skill cannot be purchased; only you can give this meaningful touch.

Most spouses do not want to hurt their partner's feelings by saying something is lacking. To avoid an argument, they remain silent. This can lead to an eventual separation or infidelity. Touching is obviously not just about sex. Touch should be something you practice daily. The five most-desired touches are hugs and kisses, massage, playful touch or tickling, foreplay and sexual touch.

Hugs and kissing are the little touches we often take for granted, but they carry your love through into eternity. It is mind-blowing that this one act costs you nothing, yet so many fail to do it. Practicing hugging every morning will considerably improve your relationship. It is free and given from the heart.

Massaging your partner and knowing how to touch properly is a learned skill that must be practiced over and over. You can only be good at what you spend your time practicing. If you paid for a massage and only got half of your body massaged, you probably would never make another appointment at that place again because it left you feeling unbalanced. A massage should leave you feeling balanced and complete. Take the time to learn the skill of touch.

It's interesting to know, some reasons infidelity occurs, cost you nothing to learn. Touching skills are obtained by your desire to learn, and your willingness to improve yourself and your relationship.

Beyond the benefits for specific conditions or diseases, many enjoy the results of massage therapy. It often produces feelings of caring, comfort, and connection. Relaxation is as important as playtime; it aids in strengthening the marriage bond and contributes to keeping healthy. One of the ways to relax is to slow down and become intentional with your time. Here are some ways you can touch and reconnect as a couple.

- A good foot massage before bed will help the body and mind relax.

- A warm towel on the back of the neck is soothing.

- Massaging the shoulders and arms help ease away stress.

Massaging Your Partner

The skin is the largest organ on your body, and physical touch is an essential need. The human need for touch begins at birth and is created for your safety and comfort. Hugs fill you with confidence and confirm, you're a couple. Your need for touch never goes away; you cannot live effectively without it. A relationship without intimacy is a lonely place. Do not get it twisted, sex does not equal intimacy. It helps you feel good about yourself and demonstrates your love.

Massage is experienced by many people from birth to death. When a baby is still in the mother's womb, they can feel the effects of massage touch. People on their death beds are massaged for the calming results they receive from the soothing touch and the closeness.

In massage therapy, understanding the differences between *Sensual and Sensuous Touch* in humans brings awareness of the need for touch. From the beginning of time, all living humans and creatures need physical touch. You may say, you are too busy or you're too shy to interconnect through touch, therefore, that leaves your partner "touch starved." You do not want your spouse deprived of something only you can provide.

Numerous studies have shown that a woman's physical need is to be touched and held. It is also important to know that women need a minimum, of *eight to ten* meaningful touches a day to stay emotionally and physically healthy. Men also benefit and are comforted through touch from their spouse after a stressful day or event. A loving touch is often welcomed by the receiver.

Massage therapy is a sensuous (affecting the senses), pleasing experience. The terms sensual and sensuous share the root sens- which means to arouse the senses. Sensual has been associated with gratifying sexual senses. Sensuous is relating to the senses instead of the intellect without the sexual undertone. We now associate something that is sensuous with pleasure to the mind or body through the senses.

Touch is the most meaningful of all our senses. Now is the time for you to be sensual in your touch with one another. Offering your spouse, a massage that you provide brings you closer. Explore and practice ways to give and receive mind and body refreshing, neck, shoulder, back and foot massages. These areas are typically the most common places to be tense, when stress is present. Massage is particularly helpful in managing this type of stress.

Begin by preparing a warm, fragrant bath or shower for the ultimate relaxation interval. The warm water will calm and relax the muscles. This is an activity you can do together, to conserve water of course! Make it special for the two of you. Take your time, use the *good* towels, the *bubbles*, light the *candles* and turn on the *music*. Take out those gifts you have been waiting to use for a special occasion; this is it!

Create your calming space with comfortable pillows, scented candles, flower petals, and relaxing music; without words which create distraction. Set aside this time for you, no cell phones, TV or other electronic distractions. Music stimulates the production of serotonin. This is one of the "feel-good" chemicals in the body that helps you relax. Keep the lights low or use candles to give the place a spa-like ambiance. Another hormone responsible for sleep and relaxation is melatonin. This is released when you are in a darker environment.

Add a relaxing aroma with scented candles, made with natural ingredients (not the paraffin-based ones that release carcinogenic toxins) and essential oils like lavender, lemongrass or jasmine.

Most importantly, relax, enjoy the journey, and focus on your partner. Be in the moment, be present. Enjoy the experience as you focus on each other.

Essential Oil Caution

Essential oils or aromatherapy or volatile oils (highly fragrant liquid components of aromatic plants, trees, and grasses) enter the bloodstream through the skin. Never apply them directly to the skin. Dilute in a carrier oil and first test on the wrist and watch for any skin irritation.

Do not massage when there is a condition present and massage would cause harm to the body.

Simple Rules

The massage should not be painful. It should feel pleasant. So be sure to check in occasionally to find out if the pressure is comfortable. Do not massage anything that feels bony. Bones do not relax. They also tend to be sensitive to pain. Everything you massage should feel relatively soft.

If you have tried to give a massage and by the time your partner felt relaxed, your hands and arms ached, no fun at all! If you keep these simple principles in mind, you will be able to give a relaxing massage without feeling worn-out:

- Keep your shoulders relaxed
- Keep your back straight and avoid bending excessively
- Relax your hands between each movement
- Use a slow, even pace
- Use your thumbs as little as possible

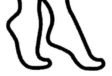

Foot Massage

There's science behind the widespread use of massage; particularly foot massage; during foreplay. According to Yasuko Kawamura; a California-based author and licensed massage therapist; states that massage increases the production of

Oxytocin. This naturally-occurring chemical is also known as the "bonding" or "cuddling" hormone. It boosts the sex drive and further increases your desire to be touched. However, foot massage doesn't have to be sexual, all the time.

A good foot massage requires focus. Imagine foot massage as an act of transferring and bringing energy and relaxation to your spouse. You won't be able to do this if you are full of negativity or not in the mood to give a massage.

A healing touch only comes from a mind entirely focused on positive things. Never give a massage if you think it is a burden or a way to release your stress. Clear your mind. Connect with your lover by breathing together. This is easily done by putting your hands on theirs and match your breathing during the session.

- When applying pressure on the soles or arches of the feet, use the "thumb-over-thumb" technique.

- Keep your back straight and let your partner's feet rest on a pillow to give you easier access.

- Use your body weight when applying pressure on the feet, especially when you are extending massage strokes up to the calves. This will lift the pressure off your fingers/hands and prevent strain injuries.

- Keep your thumbs in a hook shape when working on the feet. Using straight thumbs when providing massage strokes will cause pain in your hands.

There is nothing more relaxing than soaking your feet in a warm foot bath right before the massage. You can make an excellent foot soak with warm water in a small tub; add flower petals, a few marbles, bath salt and essential oil.

If you prefer a cleansing foot bath, simply squeeze 1/2 of a lime in a basin of warm water and essential oil, and then soak your feet. After the soak, take the other half of the lime and scrub it on the bottoms of your feet. This is a good way to remove toxins and soften your feet before the massage.

- Lift the foot in your hands, starting at the base or heel of the foot; gently pull your hands toward the toes.

- Clasp your hands around the foot and pull gently like you are milking the foot.

- Next, place your fingers down and around the Achilles heel and rub this area to help your partner relax. Circle your thumbs around the ankle bone to give it some love.

- Slide your thumb up the ball of the foot and press down gently on the sole of the foot up and under the toes. Make small circles with your thumb under the toes for ultimate pleasure.

- Then clasp the foot firmly in both hands, slowly squeeze the foot while moving your hand to the toes to complete the greatest foot massage ever!

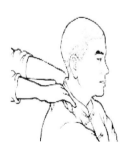

Shoulders and Neck

Movements for the shoulders and neck. Do these while your partner sits upright in a chair or on a pillow below you. The shoulder muscles are called the "trapezius" muscle. Many call them "traps" because this is where most of us trap our stress and tension.

The 1st move is a simple compression movement that uses the forearms. Stand behind your partner and rest your forearms on the top of their shoulders as close to the neck as possible (figure 1). Keep your palms down so the fleshy part of your forearm lies on the muscle.

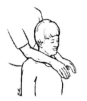

Figure 1

Let your weight fall straight down onto their shoulders toward their back. Be careful not push them too hard and do not lean on their head. Hold this position for several seconds and take some good cleansing breaths together.

Slowly lift your arms and move them down the shoulder about an inch. Let your weight fall through your arms again. Repeat this move several times. As soon as you start to feel the bony part of their shoulder under your forearm stop. Bring your forearms to the starting position and repeat the move again. This forearm compression is simple to do and it feels fabulous.

Now, move to the side of your partner for the 2nd move. Feel the tip of the shoulder with your fingers. It will feel hard and bony. Move your fingers toward the neck until you feel soft muscle under your fingers. Place your thumbs on that spot (figure 2). Put one thumb on top of the other for reinforcement — each thumb will be doing just half the work. Press straight down with the thumbs. You will be pressing on the trapezius muscle again. Press down slowly, then hold the thumbs in the muscle for a couple of seconds and then slowly ease off the pressure. Move one thumb width towards the neck and repeat the compression. You should be able to do four to six compressions before you reach the neck.

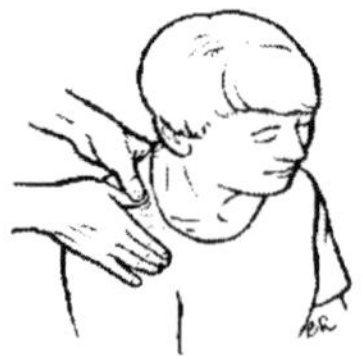

Figure 2

Once you reach the neck, move your thumbs back to the starting position and repeat this move. Go to the other side of your partner and repeat these compressions on the other shoulder.

For this 3rd amazing move, you will have to stand behind your partner. Place your hands over each shoulder (figure 3) as close to the neck as possible. Squeeze the trapezius between the fingertips and the heel of the hand. Keep your thumb beside your index finger so that it stays out of the way.

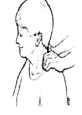

Figure 3

Hold the squeeze for a couple of seconds and then slowly release your grip. Move out a little toward the shoulders and repeat. You should be able to get three or four squeezes in before you run out of muscle. Be sure that you have the whole muscle in your hand so that you don't pinch the skin. Do not put your fingers too far around the front of the neck. You do not want to choke your partner.

In the back of the neck, you have extensor muscles that hold the head upright. Because of poor posture and extended periods of sitting at computers, these muscles can become very tight, tender and achy.

In the 4ᵗʰ move, massage the neck extensors. Stand to the side of your partner, if you are standing on the right side, make a C-shape with your left hand. Place this hand over the back of the neck. Press gently into the sides of the neck with your fingers and thumbs (figure 4).

Figure   4

With gentle pressure, do a large circular kneading action with your hand. This movement may remind you of picking a dog up by the back of the neck.

Do several circles in one spot and then move up or down the neck and repeat. Massage the length of the neck.

Be careful don't pinch the skin on the back of the neck. Roll the skin with your fingers instead of sliding over the skin, this way you won't burn or irritate the skin.

Lastly, do a little kneading to the base of the skull. This is where the extensor muscles attach to the skull. To do this, cup your hand around the base of the skull. (figure 5)

Gently rest your free hand on your partner's forehead to support the head. Now move the fingers in a small circular motion, pressing into the skull as you knead. Do six to eight little circles.

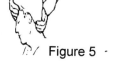

Figure 5

- Repeat the kneading action. Do several sets of this movement.

- To do the other side of the skull, move to the opposite side of your partner.

Finish the massage with several gentle strokes down the scalp and back.

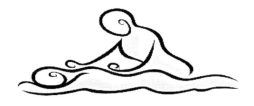

Back Massage

- Use a stable, hard surface in your home, have your loved one lay face down on their stomach.

- Place towels, blankets or another type of soft material to increase their comfort during the massage.

- Begin by applying massage lotion or oil into your hands. Start by lightly spreading the lotion/oil evenly across their back. Using the palms of your hands with your fingers together, one hand on each side of the spine, make a figure eight motion to make sure you cover the entire back. Gradually increase the amount of pressure you're applying as you continue the back rub.

- Move into your next gliding stroke by firmly moving up the back, to the shoulder and down the back again. Use your body weight to create additional pressure. Do this in a tender, fluid motion without removing your hands from your partner's body.

- If you want to go deeper with each gliding stroke, use your knuckles. Be careful not to press on bony structures, like the spine or shoulder blades.

- Apply more pressure to the muscles along each side of the spine.

- Because the shoulders are one area of the body where tension is held, be sure to apply pressure to that area. Grab the upper shoulder muscle and apply varying amounts of pressure, depending on the comfort level of the person that is getting massaged.

- Finish up the massage by returning to the initial figure eight stroke.

- Repeat several times for maximum relief from standing, sitting, driving and many everyday functions.

- You can complete and enhance this massage by placing a warm towel over the entire back as they continue to relax.

After your massage, enjoy a nice refreshing beverage, infused water is a great choice. Massages are a great way to relax and rejuvenate. By taking some extra time to give and receive massage from your spouse is pure bliss. The stress levels will be lower, your skin will feel smoother and your muscles will perform better. There are many benefits to gain by this one act of service for each other. Enjoy your time of reconnecting, now that the kids are grown.

COUPLES, REMEMBER THIS:
LOVE IS THE HEALER. IF YOU DO NOT KNOW WHERE TO PUT YOUR HANDS, AT LEAST LOVE. LOVE IS THE MOTHER OF ALL HEALING ENERGIES.

Headache and Stress Relief

Relief for stress and tension headaches, massage the following areas:

- Sides of the spine, at the base of the neck.
- The raised spot in the middle of your neck.
- Sides of the neck at the base of the skull.
- Bony part of the temples.
- Top of the ear.
- The boney spot behind the ear.
- The bridge of the nose between your eyes.
- Beneath the eyebrows in the center.
- Half an inch above the eyebrows in a circular motion.
- In the middle of the forehead, the third eye with fingers in circles.
- The web space between the thumb and index fingers, slow circles.
- The side of the spine mid-neck.
- The ridge between the shoulders and the base of the neck.

Summary

The purpose of this book is to provide couples with knowledge and awareness of reconnecting by means of massage touch. Personal touch is powerful for the empty nesters who find themselves in that silent space in the house. Now is the time to fill your space and rekindle the fire of your romance. Using massage therapy is one tool that is enjoyable, easy to perform and inexpensive, while providing many benefits for both of you. Performing these moves does not take a lot of additional time; most sessions can be done in less than ten minutes. Reconnect with your spouse, your lover, your friend and share this time in your lives together and make it better than ever! Enjoy every moment!

About the Author

Angela Dunston Thomas resides in the West Atlanta Metro area, with her husband Alan. They have three adult daughters and six grandchildren from Pre-K to College. They actively serve and worship in the community. She has worked as a Board Certified Therapeutic Massage Therapist in Georgia for the last ten years. Previous experience includes Day Spas, Sports Health Facilities, Chiropractic Offices as well as the owner of Angela's Therapeutic Massage. In addition to massage therapy, she has been employed in public education for nearly 30 years and presently works in the local public-school system. She shares her life with some amazing people who inspire her by living out loud by their actions and not mere words alone. Angela and Alan enjoy traveling, photography, and cooking with family and friends.

For additional information or appointments:

Email: aythomas27@gmail.com

Angela Thomas, L.M.T., MT005039, NCBTMB #551571-08

Instagram: romance_angel13

References

Anderson, N. T. (2006). *The bondage breaker*. Eugene, OR: Harvest
House Publishers.

Carlyle, T. (n.d.). BrainyQuote. Retrieved from
https://www.brainyquote.com/authors/thomas_carlyle

Connor, L. (2015, November 2015). Divorce rates at lowest for 40 years
except for over-50 'silver splitters.' *Mirror*. Retrieved from
https://www.mirror.co.uk/news/uk-news/divorce-rates-lowest-40-
years-6887383

Dobson, J. (n.d.). Children are not casual guests in our home. Retrieved
from http://www.quotes-inspirational.com/quote/children-not-
casual-guests-our-210/

Douglass, F. (n.d.). It is easier to build strong children than to repair
broken men... Retrieved from http://www.quotes-
inspirational.com/quote/easier-build-strong-children-repair-85/

God will protect me quotes. (n.d.). SearchQuotes. Retrieved from
www.searchquotes.com/search/God_Will_Protect_Me/

Graham, A. D. (n.d.). Live without pretending... Retrieved from
http://www.searchquotes.com/quotation/Live_without_pretending,

 Love without depending, Listen without defending, Speak wi
 thout_offending/245182/

Fincham, F. D., & Beach, S. R. H. (2014). I say a little prayer for you:

Praying for partner increases commitment in romantic

relationships. *Journal of Family Psychology, 28*(5), 587-593. doi:

10.1037/a0034999

Frederick, R. (2016, October 19). *The '15 second kiss' experiment.*

Retrieved from https://fiercemarriage.com/15-second-kiss-

experiment

Littauer, F. (2001). *Personality plus for couples: Understanding yourself*

and the one you love. Grand Rapids, MI: Baker Publishing Group.

Manger, W. (2013, May 27). 50 ways to live life to the full: From wealth

and health to love and laughter. *Mirror.* Retrieved from

https://www.mirror.co.uk/lifestyle/health/50-ways-live-life-full-

1875014

Nunes, R. A. (n.d.). Goodreads. Retrieved from

https://www.goodreads.com/quotes/63885-do-what-makes-you-

happy-be-with-who-makes-you

Phillips, M. (2000). *Married for life: Life-giving principles that make a*

marriage last. Lakewood,

CO: Marriage Ministries International.

Prather, H. (2001). AZ quotes. Retrieved from

http://www.azquotes.com/quote/235775

Ramsey, D. (2012). *Dave Ramsey's complete guide to money: The handbook of financial peace university.* Brentwood, TN: Ramsey Press.

Rutherford, M. (2014, July 20). Am I over empty nest? Who am I kidding... *The Huffington Post.* Retrieved from

https://www.huffingtonpost.com/dr-margaret-rutherford/getting-over-empty-nest-_b_5581837.html

Shanley, J. P. (n.d.). AZ quotes. Retrieved from

http://www.azquotes.com/author/18235-John_Patrick_Shanley

Swedish proverbs & sayings. (n.d.). Inspirational quotes. Retrieved from

https://www.inspirationalquotes4u.com/swedishproverbs/index.html

Van Dyke, H. (n.d.). BrainyQuote. Retrieved from
https://www.brainyquote.com/quotes/henry_van_dyke_391213